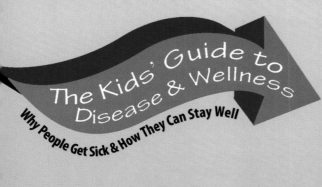

The Kids' Guide to
Disease & Wellness
Why People Get Sick & How They Can Stay Well

WHY CAN'T I BREATHE?

Kids & Asthma

Rae Simons

The Kids' Guide to Disease & Wellness:
Why People Get Sick and How They Can Stay Well
WHY CAN'T I BREATHE? KIDS & ASTHMA

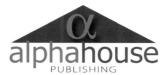

AlphaHouse Publishing
201 Harding Avenue
Vestal, NY 13850

First Printing

9 8 7 6 5 4 3 2 1

ISBN: 978-1-934970-15-7
ISBN (series): 978-1-934970-11-9
Library of Congress Control Number: 2008930673

Author: Simons, Rae

Cover design by MK Bassett-Harvey.
Interior design by MK Bassett-Harvey and Wendy Arakawa.

Printed in India by International Print-O-Pac Limited

 An ISO 9001 Company

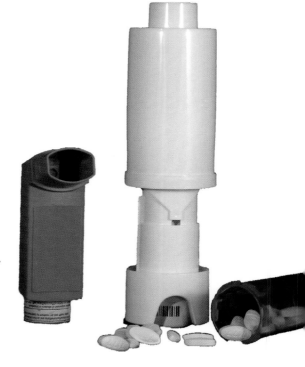

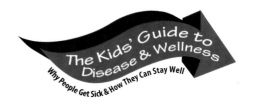

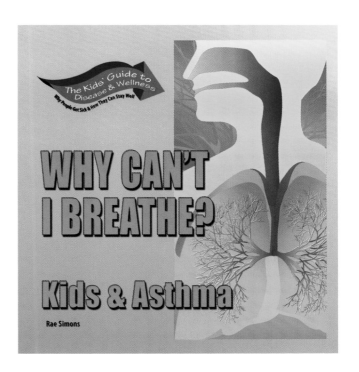

by Rae Simons

Series List

Introduction

According to a recent study reported in the Virginia Henderson International Nursing Library, kids worry about getting sick. They worry about AIDS and cancer, about allergies and the "super-germs" that resist medication. They know about these ills—but they don't always understand what causes them or how they can be prevented.

Unfortunately, most 9- to 11–year–olds, the study found, get their information about diseases like AIDS from friends and television; only 20 percent of the children interviewed based their understanding of illness on facts they had learned at school. Too often, kids believe urban legends, schoolyard folktales, and exaggerated movie plots. Oftentimes, misinformation like this only makes their worries worse. The January 2008 *Child Health News* reported that 55 percent of all children between 9 and 13 "worry almost all the time" about illness.

This series, **The Kids' Guide to Disease and Wellness**, offers readers clear information on various illnesses and conditions, as well as the immunizations that can prevent many diseases. The books dispel the myths with clearly presented facts and colorful, accurate illustrations. Better yet, these books will help kids understand not only illness—but also what they can do to stay as healthy as possible.

—*Dr. Elise Berlan*

Just The Facts

- Asthma is a chronic disease that affects the airways to your lungs, and makes it difficult to breathe.

- Asthma is an allergy that can be passed on genetically, or stimulated by the environment.

- Inhalers, nebulizers, and steroids are all used to treat asthma symptoms. Medication is taken to prevent asthma in the first place.

- Playing wind instruments and sports can actually strengthen your lungs if you have asthma, as long as they're done with caution.

- Asthma is a global problem. No cures have been found, but medications and technology are available to help treat asthma.

What Is Asthma?

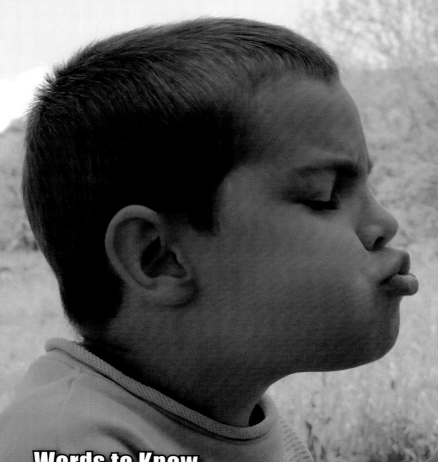

Words to Know

Chronic: having to do with something that's long-lasting and ongoing (usually a disease).

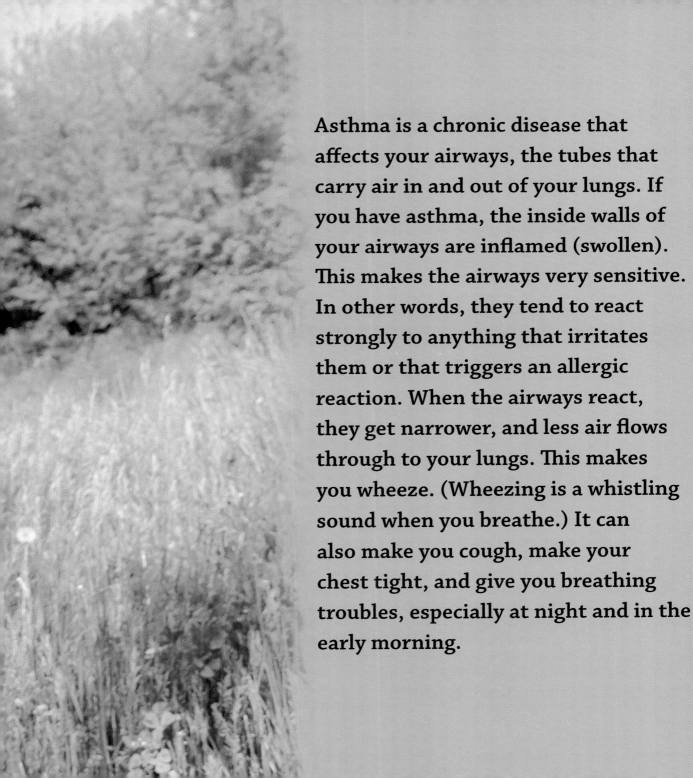

Asthma is a chronic disease that affects your airways, the tubes that carry air in and out of your lungs. If you have asthma, the inside walls of your airways are inflamed (swollen). This makes the airways very sensitive. In other words, they tend to react strongly to anything that irritates them or that triggers an allergic reaction. When the airways react, they get narrower, and less air flows through to your lungs. This makes you wheeze. (Wheezing is a whistling sound when you breathe.) It can also make you cough, make your chest tight, and give you breathing troubles, especially at night and in the early morning.

Your Respiratory System

All the cells in your body require oxygen. Without it, they couldn't move, build, grow, or turn food into energy. Without oxygen, you and your cells would die.

Oxygen comes from the air you inhale through your nose and mouth. The air flows down through the windpipe, to where the windpipe divides into two tubes that lead into the lungs. If you could see your lungs, you might think they looked like big, red sponges. Inside the spongy tissue, tubes called bronchi branch into even smaller tubes. They look like the branches of a tree.

Words to Know

Inhale: breathe in.

Exhale: breathe out.

Did You Know?

If you could spread out flat all the air sacs in an adult's lungs, they would cover an area about a third the size of a tennis court.

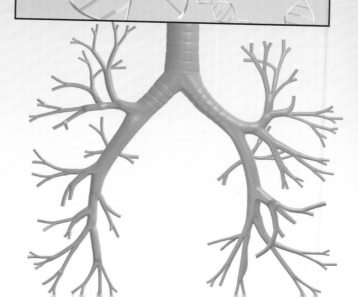

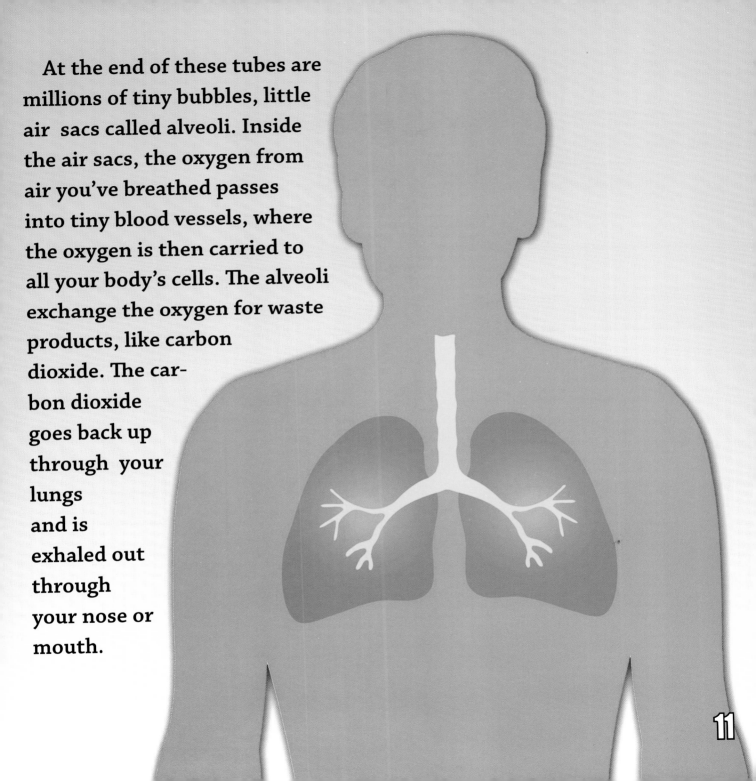

At the end of these tubes are millions of tiny bubbles, little air sacs called alveoli. Inside the air sacs, the oxygen from air you've breathed passes into tiny blood vessels, where the oxygen is then carried to all your body's cells. The alveoli exchange the oxygen for waste products, like carbon dioxide. The carbon dioxide goes back up through your lungs and is exhaled out through your nose or mouth.

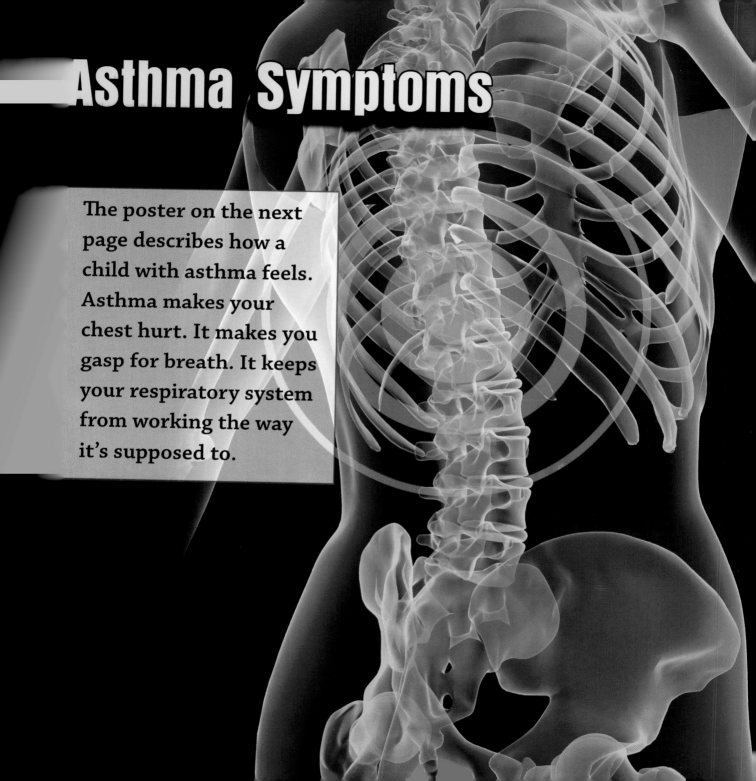

Asthma Symptoms

The poster on the next page describes how a child with asthma feels. Asthma makes your chest hurt. It makes you gasp for breath. It keeps your respiratory system from working the way it's supposed to.

"WHEN I HAVE AN ASTHMA ATTACK I FEEL LIKE A FISH WITH NO WATER."

–JESSE, AGE 5

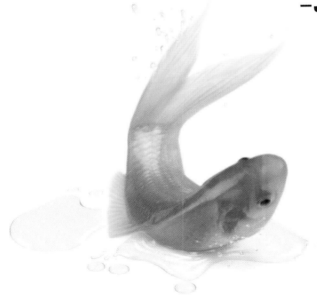

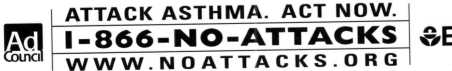

13

What Does Asthma Do Inside Your Body?

The reason why asthma makes a person gasp for breath is because of what it does to the inside of the lungs.

Words to Know

Mucus: a thick, slippery fluid produced by the linings of your nose, lungs, and throat.

14

Someone told me that if I have asthma, I won't grow as tall. Is that true?

A: No, not if your asthma is being treated by a doctor. Sometimes severe asthma can slow the onset of puberty (the stage where your body starts turning into an adult). This can mean you may get your height later than other kids your age. But so long as you do what your doctor tells you, and your asthma is under good control, your asthma won't get in the way of your growth.

During an asthma attack, the sides of the airways in your lungs swell, and the airways shrink. Less air gets in and out of your lungs. Mucus clogs up the airways even more.

15

Who Gets Asthma?

Asthma often starts in early childhood. Even babies can have asthma. It is the most common chronic disease in children. Some children outgrow asthma as they get older.

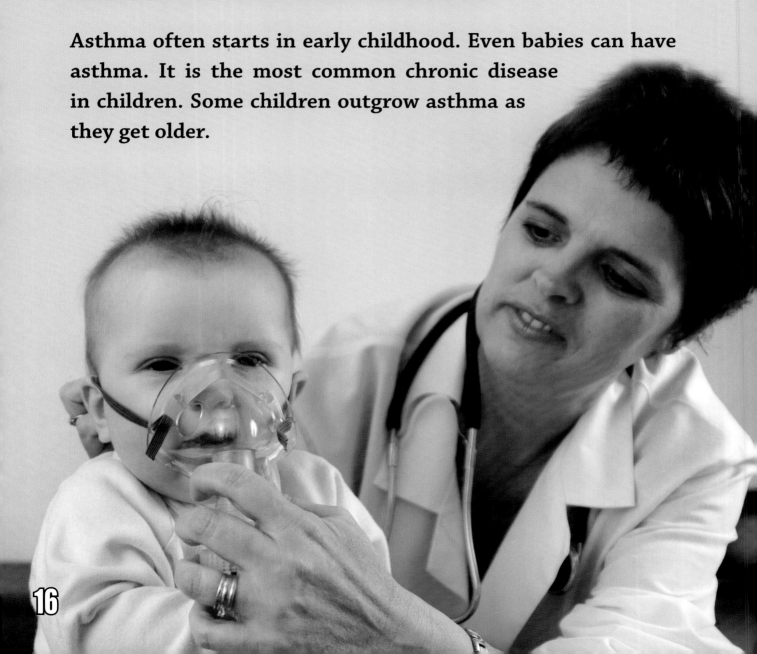

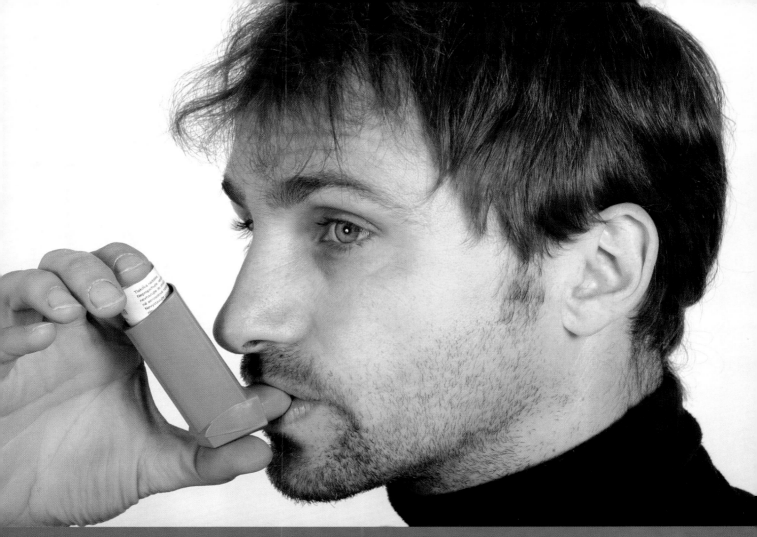

But adults get asthma, too. Around the world, about 300 million people have asthma. Asthma affects all the countries in the world, but it is more dangerous to people living in poverty. More people die from asthma in low-income countries.

Words to Know

Poverty: the condition of being poor (lacking money and/or the basic necessities of life).

17

What Causes Asthma?

Words to Know

Factors: things that help produce a result.

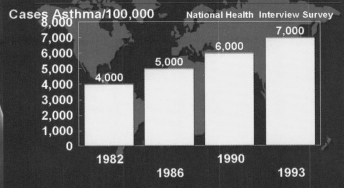

Rate of asthma in the U.S. children 0-17 years of age

Cases Asthma/100,000   National Health Interview Survey

- 8,000
- 7,000 — 7,000 (1993)
- 6,000 — 6,000 (1990)
- 5,000 — 5,000 (1986)
- 4,000 — 4,000 (1982)
- 3,000
- 2,000
- 1,000
- 0

1982 1986 1990 1993

Why asthma makes it hard to breathe

Air enters the respiratory system from the nose and mouth and travels through the bronchial tubes.

In an asthmatic person, the muscles of the bronchial tubes tighten and thicken, and the air passages become inflamed and mucus-filled, making it difficult for air to move.

In a non-asthmatic person, the muscles around the bronchial tubes are relaxed and the tissue thin, allowing for easy airflow.

Inflamed bronchial tube of an asthmatic

Normal bronchial tube

Source: American Academy of Allergy, Asthma and Immunology

Asthma is becoming more and more common. If you look at the chart to the left, you can see how the numbers of children with asthma climbed in the years between 1982 and 1993—and they have continued to climb since then. Doctors believe this is because of a number of factors. Allergies, poor indoor air quality, and pollution may all play a role.

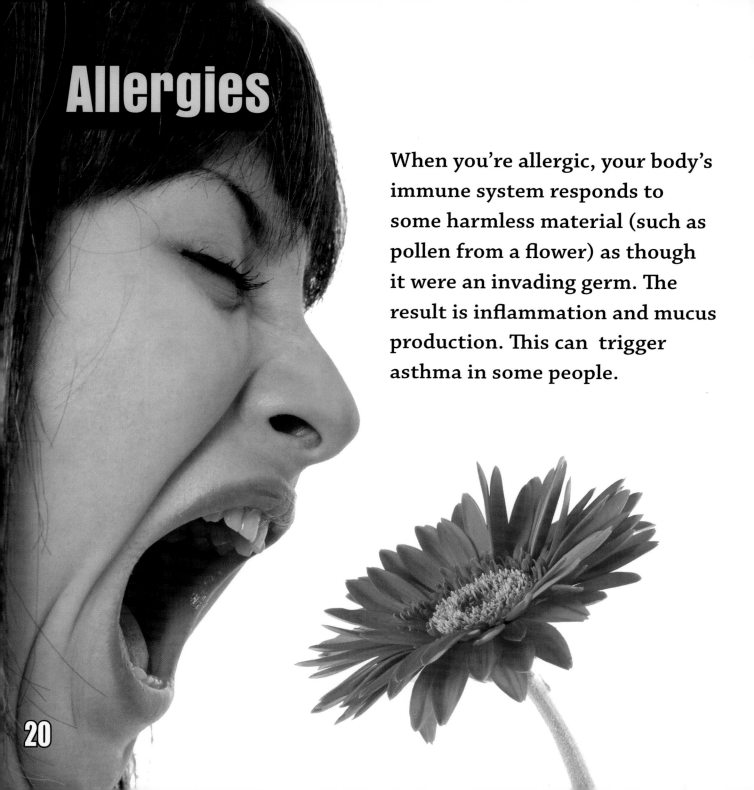

Allergies

When you're allergic, your body's immune system responds to some harmless material (such as pollen from a flower) as though it were an invading germ. The result is inflammation and mucus production. This can trigger asthma in some people.

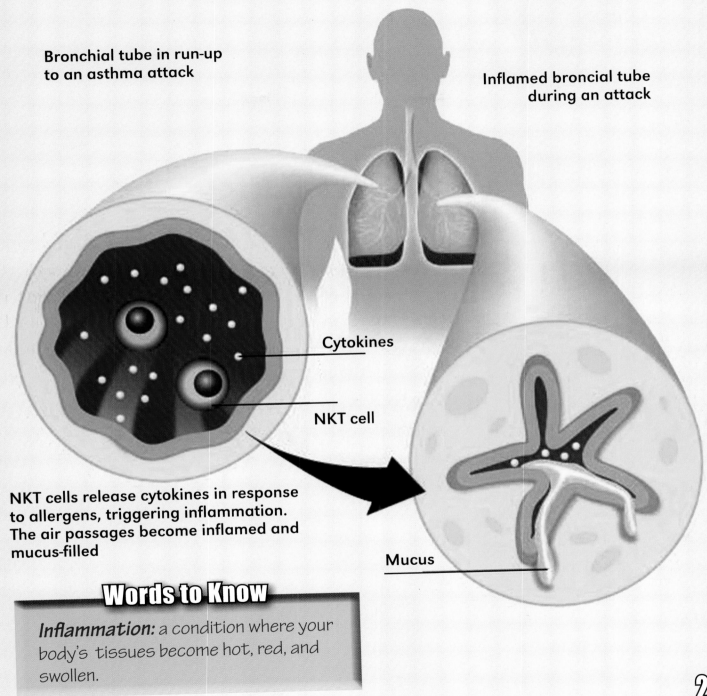

Bronchial tube in run-up to an asthma attack

Inflamed broncial tube during an attack

Cytokines

NKT cell

NKT cells release cytokines in response to allergens, triggering inflammation. The air passages become inflamed and mucus-filled

Mucus

Words to Know

Inflammation: a condition where your body's tissues become hot, red, and swollen.

21

Pollution

Pollution is what happens when we make our world dirty. Air pollution (like what's shown here) is made up of chemicals, smoke, and tiny particles.

Words to Know

Concentration: the amount of some substance per unit of another substance (such as grams per liter).

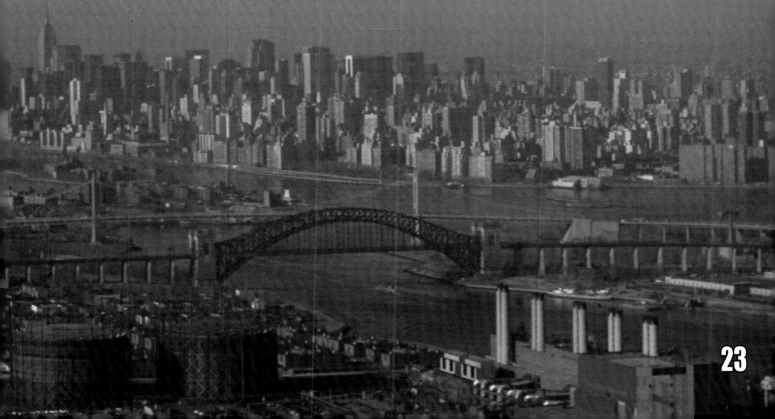

Air pollution is one of the things that can trigger asthma. Scientists have shown that air pollution from cars, factories, and power plants is a major cause of asthma attacks. Even people who don't normally have asthma can have a first attack when exposed to air that has a heavy concentration of pollution.

Secondhand Smoke

Secondhand smoke is what smokers exhale, plus any smoke from the burning end of a cigarette, cigar, or pipe. Secondhand smoke contains more than 4,000 chemicals—and none of them are good for you!

Words to Know

Irritates: causes inflammation in a body tissue (such as skin).

24

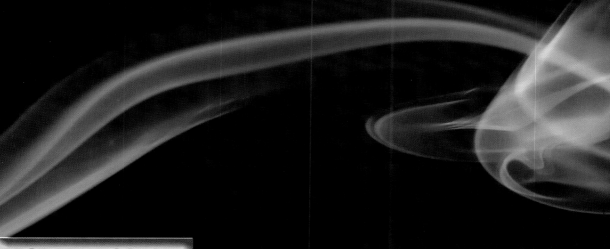

ASK THE DOCTOR

Why are childen more apt to develop asthma than adults?

A: Because children's bodies are developing rapidly, anything that gets in the way of their normal growth makes them more vulnerable to injury and illness. Also, children's airways are smaller than adults', so they have more asthma symptoms, like wheezing and shortness of breath, than adults with the same degree of asthma.

Secondhand smoke can both trigger asthma attacks AND make the attacks w Pre-school children who have never had asthma before are more apt to develop it if they are exposed to secondhand smoke Scientists believe the smoke irritates air passageways.

Genetics

Your genes are the tiny pieces of DNA (illustrated here)—and DNA is the material inside each of your body's cells that was passed down to you from your parents. Each gene contains a particular set of instructions for your cells.

Words to Know

Traits: features of an individual's nature.

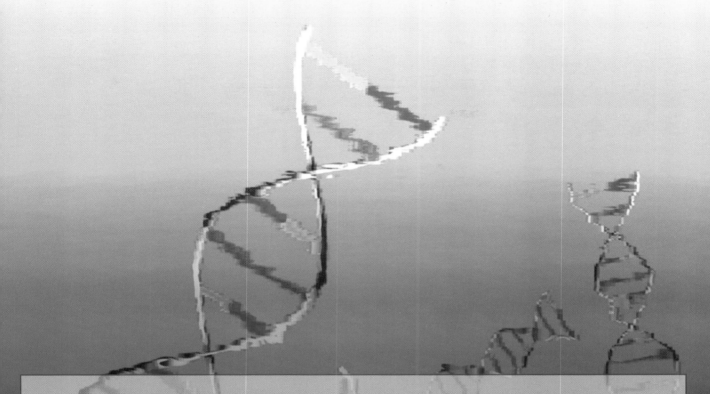

Your genes are your body's "blueprint." They are what make you have brown hair or blonde, dark skin or pale, blue eyes or brown. They also carry the instructions for other traits that can make you more likely to get a particular disease or condition.

Scientists believe that about half of all cases of asthma are linked to genetics (while the other half are caused mostly by triggers in the environment). This means if your parents and others in your family have asthma, you're more apt to have it, too.

How Do You Know If You Have Asthma?

If you have bouts of wheezing, coughing, and being short of breath, your doctor may suspect you have asthma. You'll need to have some tests to find out for sure.

These tests don't hurt. The doctor will look inside your nose and throat to see if your tissues there are inflamed. He'll listen with a stethoscope to your breathing. He may ask you to blow through a device like the one to the right, a peak flow meter.

Words to Know

Stethoscope: a device like the one around the doctor's neck to the right, used for listening to heartbeat and other body sounds.

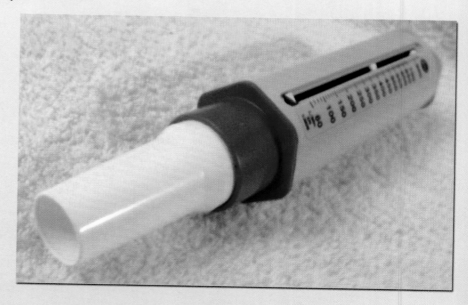

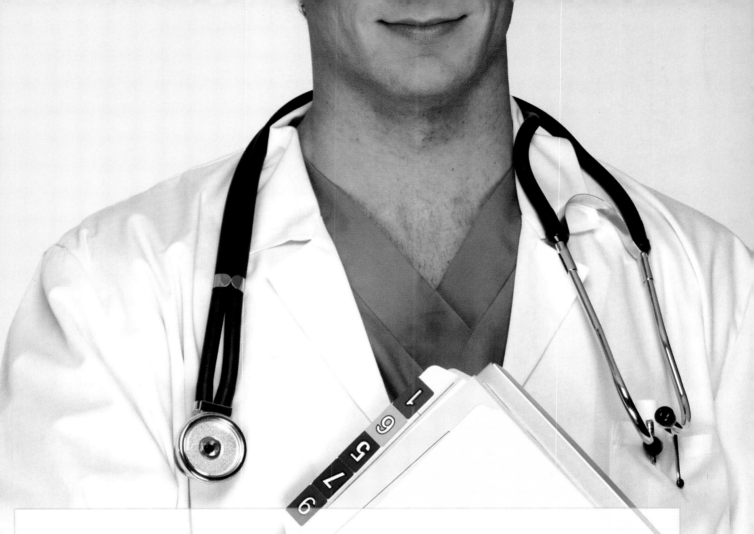

A peak flow meter like this one measures how much air flows out of your lungs when you push it out in one quick blast. Another test uses a machine called a spirometer. For this test, you take deep breaths and push them out as hard as you can into a hose. The spirometer measures how fast and how much you can breathe in and out.

29

How Is Asthma Treated?

If your doctor decides you have asthma, she will probably want you take medicine that will help you breathe better.

ASK THE DOCTOR

Can you get "high" from using an inhaler?

A: No, you can't. If you use your inhaler too often, the only thing you'll feel is a little dizzy and lightheaded. Your heart may also beat faster. But it won't make you high!

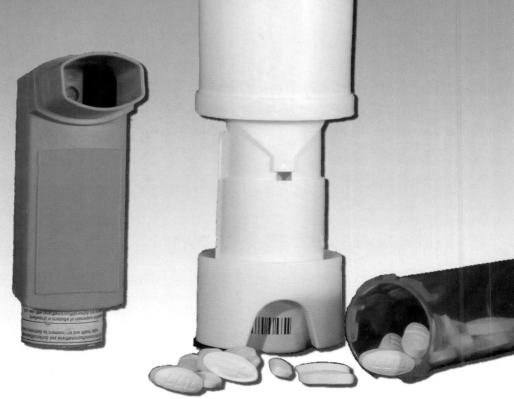

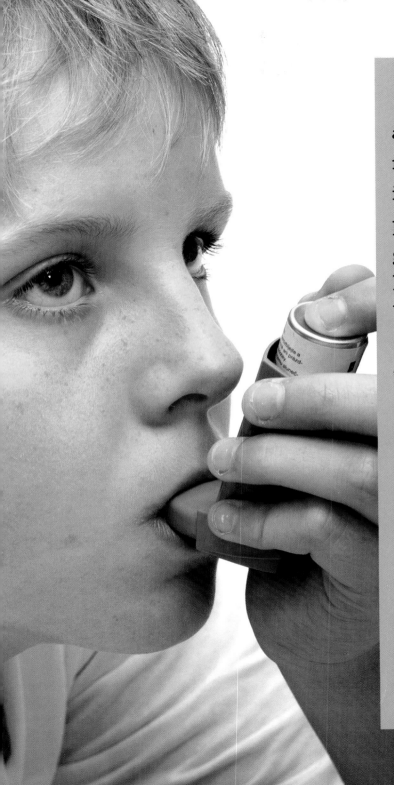

Asthma medicine comes in a few different forms. Some medicines are meant to be inhaled. These often come in packages that look like the gray and white ones on the left page. When you push a button, they release a puff of medicine that you suck into your lungs. Other asthma medications are pills you will probably need to take every day. Some medicines act quickly and provide short-term relief. Others are long-lasting and are meant to prevent asthma symptoms. Your doctor will help you decide which are best for you.

31

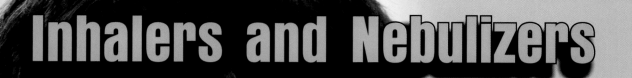

Inhalers and Nebulizers

An inhaler is shown on this page, and a nebulizer on the page to the right. Both allow you to breathe in asthma medicine. An inhaler gives a quick puff, while the nebulizer allows you to breathe the medicine steadily.

Did You Know?

Medicines like these are called bronchodilaters, because they dilate (make wider) the bronchial tubes in your lungs. They are also sometimes called "rescue" medications, because they stop an asthma attack that's in progress.

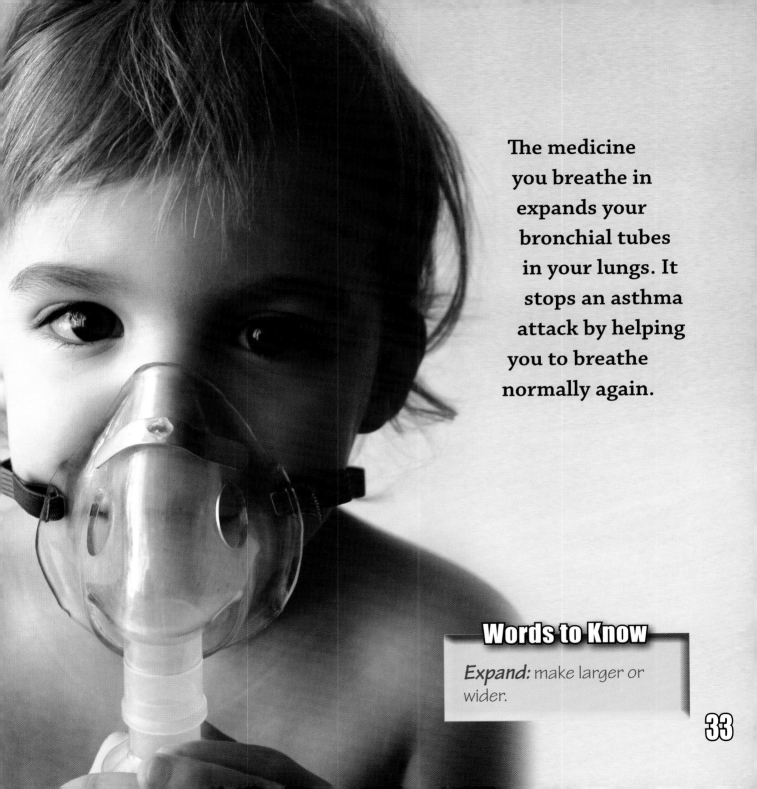

The medicine you breathe in expands your bronchial tubes in your lungs. It stops an asthma attack by helping you to breathe normally again.

Words to Know

Expand: make larger or wider.

33

Steroids

Steroids are a type of chemical that helps reduce asthma symptoms by getting rid of some of the swelling and mucus in a person's airways.

Steroids are usually inhaled, often from a package that looks like the one shown on this page. This medicine is good for preventing asthma attacks—but it won't help you when you're in the middle of one.

Words to Know

Reduce: make smaller or make happen less often.

Did You Know?

The kind of steroids used to treat asthma aren't the same as the ones used by some athletes to make their muscles larger. The steroids you take if you have asthma are safer and have few side effects. Only very small amounts are needed to reduce asthma symptoms.

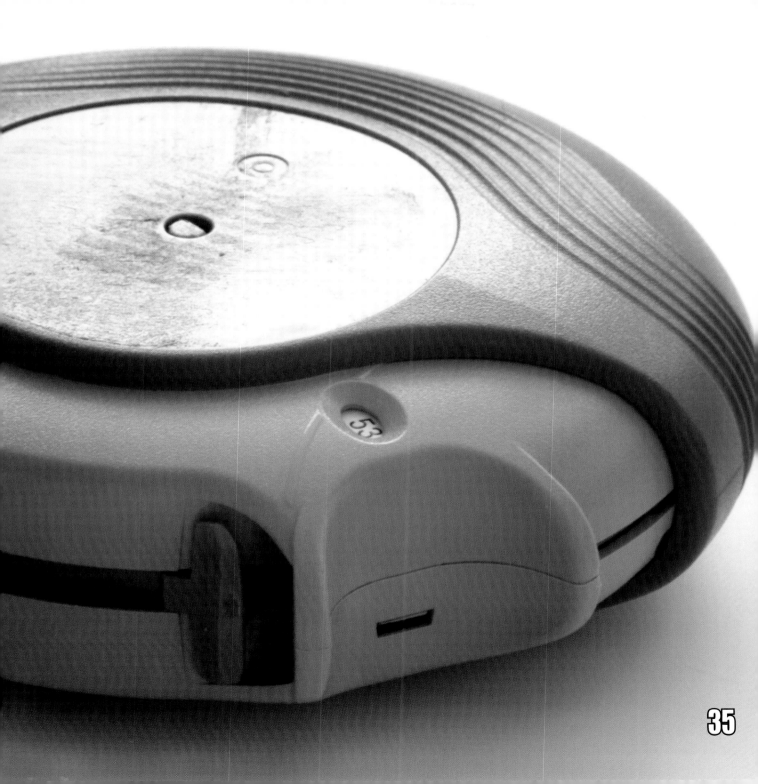

Alternative Treatments

Some people are uncomfortable with taking chemicals to treat their asthma. They may try alternative treatments instead, such as yoga (shown here) or acupuncture (shown on the next page.) Doctors agree that both of these can help reduce asthma symptoms. Yoga exercises strengthen your respiratory system and improve your lung function. Acupuncture, which involves placing needles in

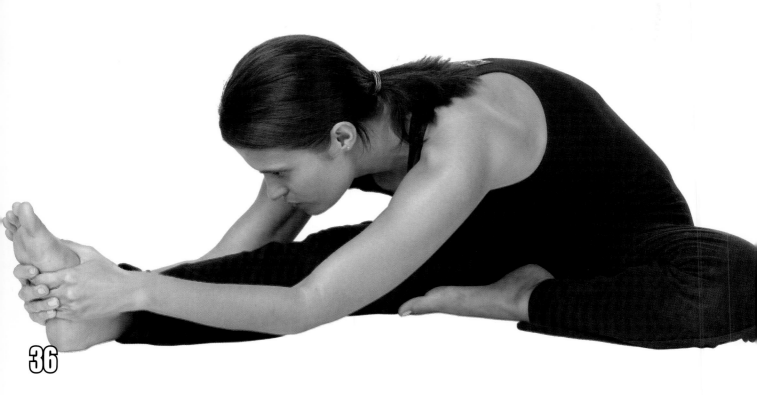

certain parts of your body (it doesn't hurt!), can also help you breathe better. Both of these techniques are based on traditional Asian medicine. While both can help prevent asthma symptoms, neither is much use when you're actually in the middle of an attack. That's why doctors recommend using these treatments along with medication as needed.

Words to Know

Alternative: allowing a choice.

Function: ability to do the job intended.

37

What Happens If You Don't Take Your Medicine?

If you find out you have asthma, it's important to take your medication. Even if you don't have an asthma attack, you may have ongoing low-level symptoms, such as chest pains, cough, and a stuffy nose. Germs can get stuck in the extra mucus in your airways and make you sick more often with colds.

Taking your medicine helps keep you healthier. It allows you to do all the things you want to without having to gasp for air.

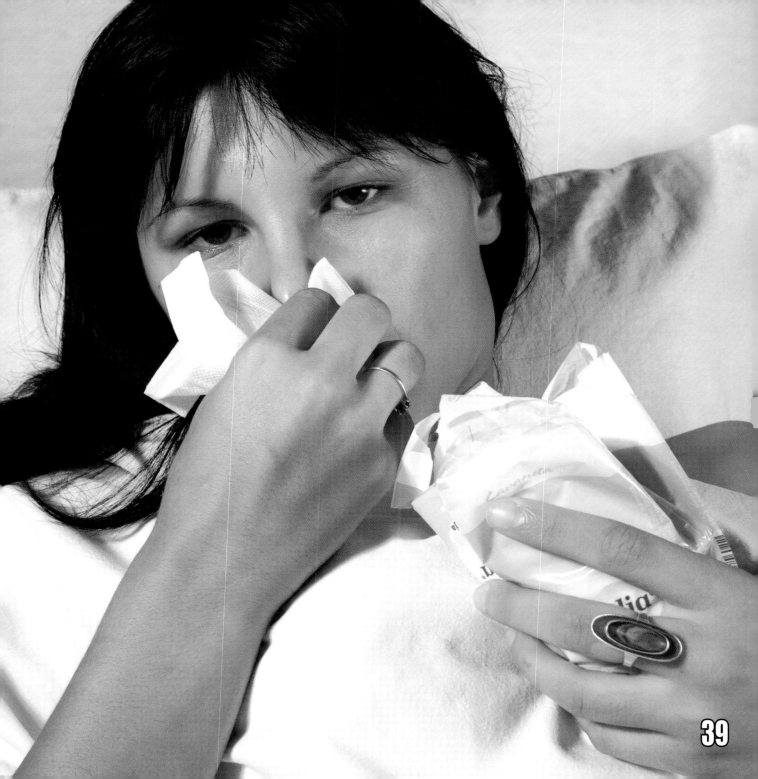

Will Having Asthma Change Your Life?

Having asthma (or any other illness) means you have to pay more attention to your body. You have to listen to the messages your body gives you. Learning to avoid the triggers that cause you to have asthma (things you're allergic to, for example, or cigarette smoke or emotional stress) can help you control your asthma symptoms better. But that doesn't mean that asthma has to control YOU!

Did You Know?

Your emotions can trigger an asthma attack. When you're upset or stressed, you are much more likely to have asthma symptoms.

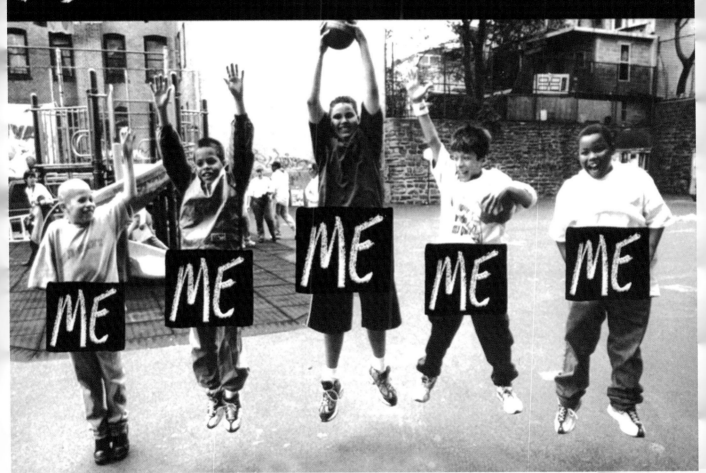

Can You Still Exercise?

If you have asthma, you may feel like you don't want to exercise. Running around makes you breathe harder, and breathing harder can sometimes trigger asthma. You may also feel like it's hard to get enough oxygen to exercise.

Did You Know?

Try to avoid exercising in air that's very cold, smoky, or polluted.

Many professional athletes have asthma. But they don't let that stop them!

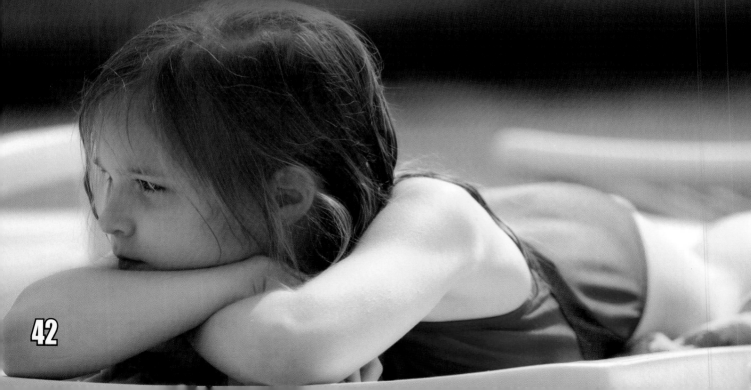

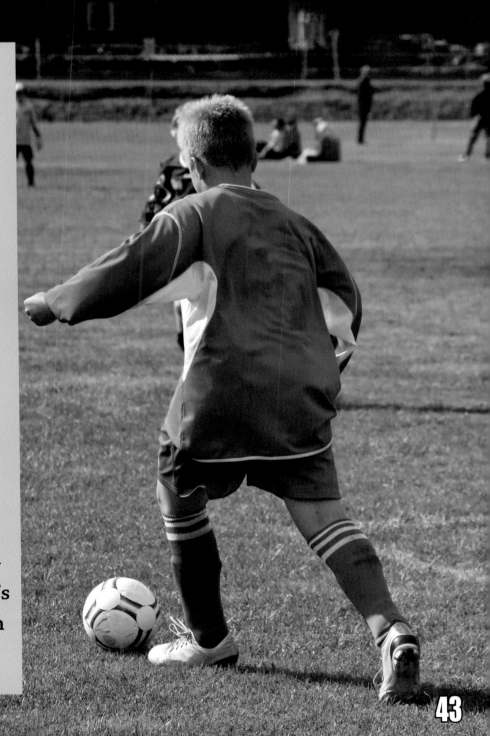

But even though asthma can make exercise harder, that doesn't mean you should stop exercising! Doctors say that exercise is actually good for asthma because it makes your lungs stronger—so you're less apt to have asthma symptoms. Just be careful to take your asthma medicine and bring your rescue inhaler with you when you exercise. Pay attention to what your body's saying, so you can learn to avoid attacks.

Can You Play a Musical Instrument?

Playing a wind instrument like a clarinet, flute, trumpet, or recorder can be hard if you can't breathe. If you have asthma, you may feel as though you shouldn't bother trying to play one of these instruments.

But remember, you don't need to let asthma control your life! Learning to play a wind instrument can improve your lung function. It can teach you how to breathe more efficiently. It can actually help you avoid asthma attacks.

So if you're musical, a wind instrument might be exactly right for you!

Did You Know?

Some doctors are teaching children to play recorders as a way to help them learn how to breathe through an asthma attack.

Because asthma attacks are scary, children may breathe faster and make their symptoms worse. Learning to play a recorder helps them learn how to stay calm and focused on their breathing during an asthma attack.

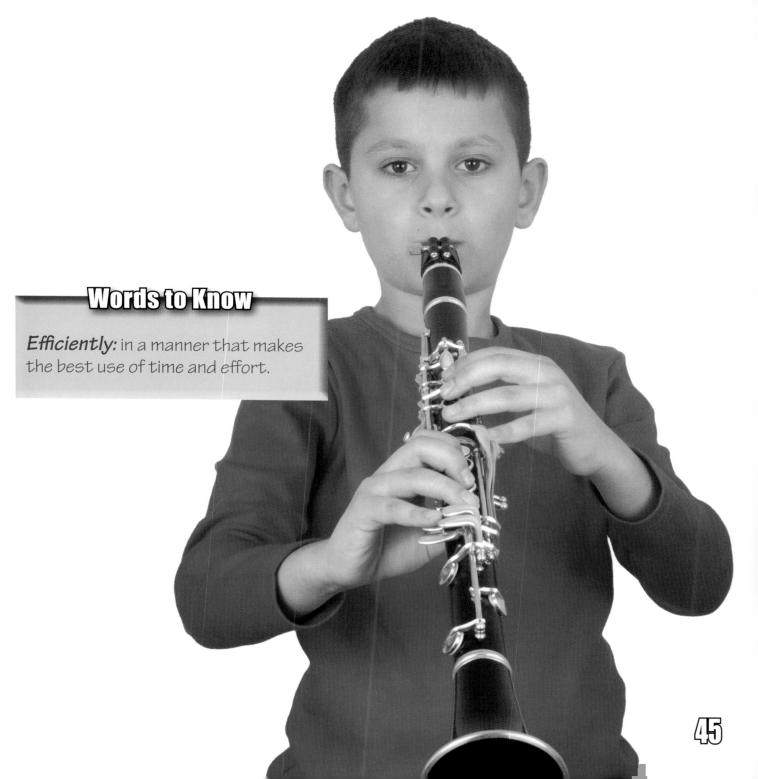

Efficiently: in a manner that makes the best use of time and effort.

What Is the World Doing About Asthma?

As asthma becomes more and more common, people are working together to find ways to fight this disease. Teaching people more about what asthma is and how it's treated can help kids who may have this condition without even knowing it. Raising money for research will help scientists understand better what causes asthma and how it can be prevented.

Words to Know

Awareness: having knowledge about something.

ASTHMA

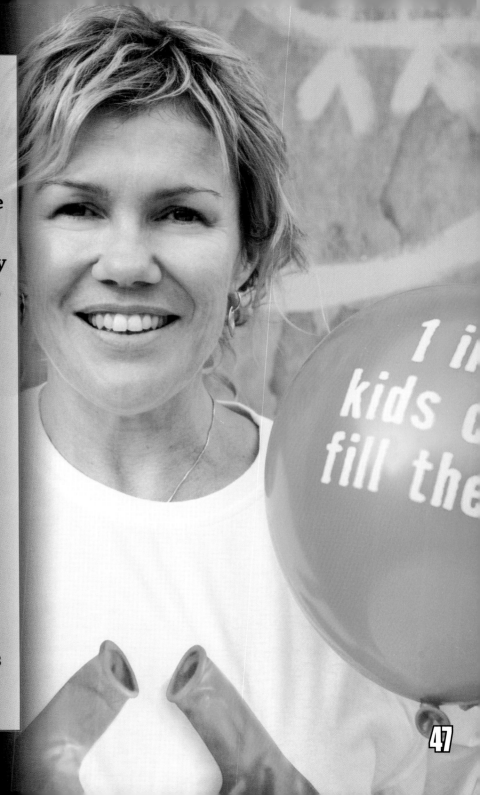

In New Zealand, for example, television star Robyn Malcolm is giving her support to asthma awareness by backing the Asthma and Respiratory Foundation's Balloon Day campaign. The event also raises funds to support research that benefits children with asthma. (Robyn's balloon shown here says, "1 in 4 kids can't fill these.") Robyn doesn't have asthma herself, but she grew up with two younger sisters who did. She knows how important it is to help children find better ways to live with asthma.

47

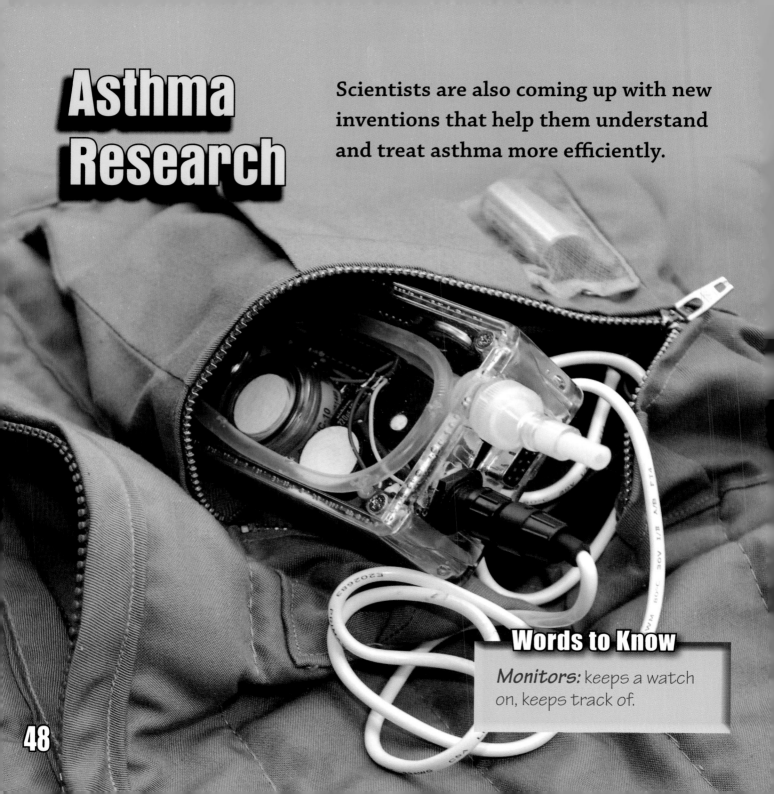

Asthma Research

Scientists are also coming up with new inventions that help them understand and treat asthma more efficiently.

Words to Know

Monitors: keeps a watch on, keeps track of.

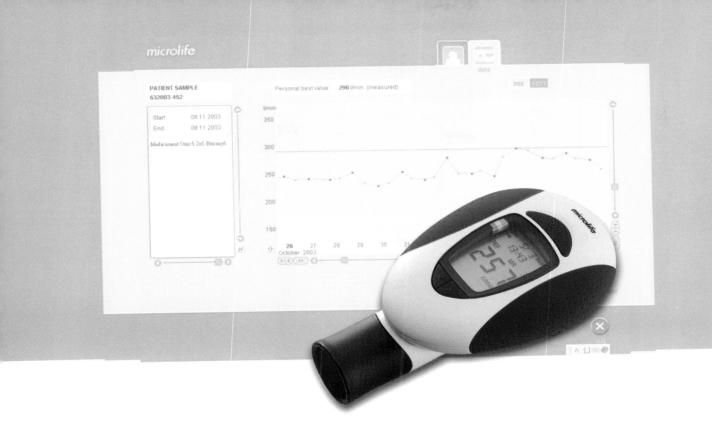

For example, a sensor system (shown to the left) that fits in the pocket monitors the air around people who have asthma. Researchers can then see what was in the air when a person has an asthma attack. This may help them understand better how to prevent attacks.

The digital asthma monitor shown above allows you to monitor your asthma by measuring your lung function. This lets you to know if you need to adjust your behavior or your medication to prevent an asthma attack.

Organizations

Because asthma is such a big problem for so many children and adults, people have joined together in organizations to fight this condition. Here are just a few of the most important ones:

- World Lung Foundation
- World Allergy Organization
- Global Alliance Against Chronic Respiratory Disease (GARD)
- Asthma UK
- American Lung Association

Words to Know

Organizations: groups of people working together with a plan to achieve a particular goal.

Did You Know?

GARD is a part of the World Health Organization (WHO). It helps individuals and asthma organizations in many countries work together.

GLOBAL ASTHMA RATES

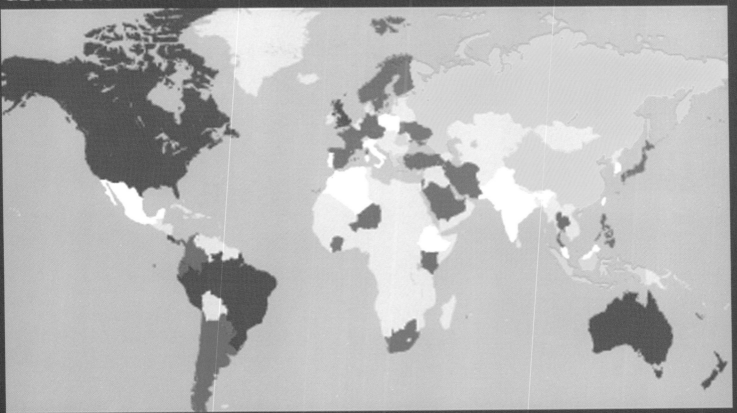

Percentage of the population affected.

10.1 +	5.1 - 7.5	0 - 2.5
7.6 - 10.0	2.5 - 5.0	No standardised data avialable

The map above shows why organizations around the world are working on this problem—because asthma circles the globe. The countries colored green and red are where asthma is most common.

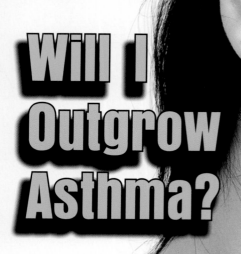

Will I Outgrow Asthma?

Doctors know that asthma symptoms get better sometimes and even disappear, but they have no way to predict when or if that will happen. They think it depends partly on how old you were when you got asthma and how bad your symptoms were.

About half the young children who have mild asthma will have no symptoms by the time they reach their mid-teens. Many years of treatment (taking asthma medication) can make asthma symptoms disappear altogether. Some people, however, will have relapses in their 20s or later in adulthood. And people who get asthma for the first time when they are older are more likely to have it for the rest of their lives.

Words to Know

Relapses: the returns of disease symptoms.

Can Asthma Be Prevented?

Scientists are trying to find ways to keep so many people from developing asthma. One of the things they're looking into is diet.

Studies have shown that teens who don't eat many fruits and vegetables are more likely to have asthma. Other research indicates that the kinds of fruit and vegetables that are brightly colored may contain chemicals and vitamins that help prevent asthma.

Scientists aren't sure yet exactly what the connection is between diet and asthma—but it never hurts to eat more fruit and vegetables!

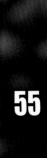

Real Kids

Leon has had asthma since he was five months old. Thanks to the medication he still uses and always carries with him, his asthma is now under control. Leon loves ballroom dancing. He's won nine gold medals and was first in all the categories in which he participated. He also plays rugby and is looking forward to going to his first Boy Scouts camp soon. He's not letting asthma get in the way of his life.

(Read more about Leon and other children with asthma who live in Cape Town, South Africa, at www.health24.com/medical/Condition_centres/777-792-800-1536,31578.asp.)

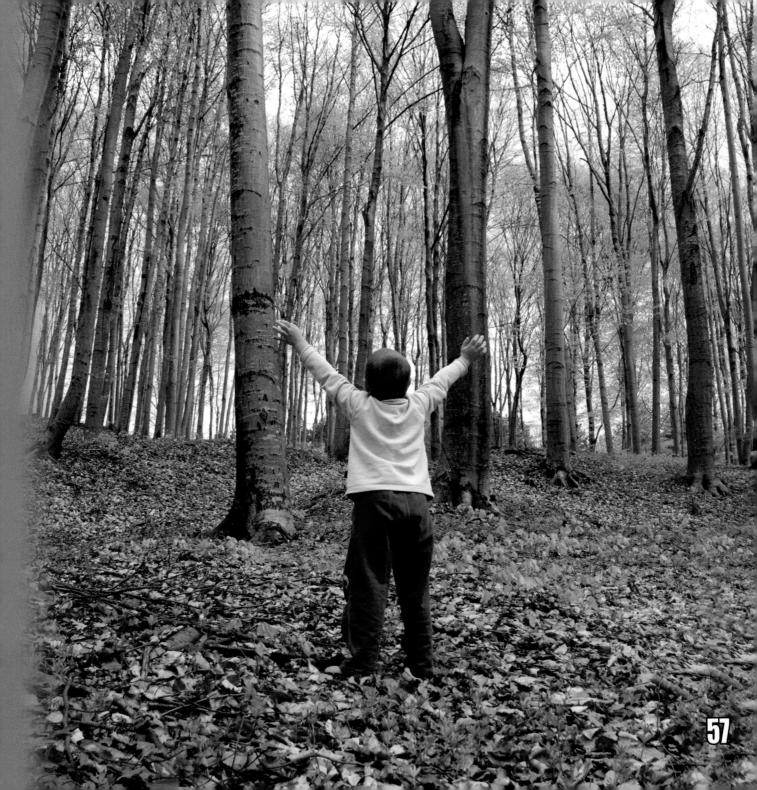

Another Real Kid

When you look at Katie, you don't see a "sick" child. When you hear about her great ability to play hockey or soccer, you don't hear about the medications she has to take several times a day so she can play. When you know about her good marks in school, you don't know about the war going on inside her body.

Katie has asthma and . . . she has to battle for what most children take for granted—to be able to breathe. There are times when each breath is a struggle and being afraid is normal.

Katie is doing her part—taking her medications (even when she sometimes wishes she didn't have to), avoiding her asthma triggers (like not being able have a cat and being an amazing athlete (even though there are times when her chest hurts a lot.) Does it all make a difference? When we asked Katie this question, her answer included this example: "Some winters I miss at least 14 days of school. This year, I've missed only three so far." For Katie, it's all about being able to be a regular, active kid who loves to play sports.

(The Lung Association, an organization working to fight asthma, tells about Katie on its Web site, www.lung.ca/diseases-maladies/asthma-asthme/faces-visages/katie_e.)phpdirty.

Find Out More

These Web sites will tell you more about asthma:

Asthma: American Lung Association
www.lungusa.org/site/c.dvLUK9O0E/b.33276

The Asthma Society of Canada
www.asthma.ca/

Asthma UK
www.asthma.org.uk/

CDC Asthma
ww.cdc.gov/asthma/

GINA: Global Initiative for Asthma
www.ginasthma.org/Guidelineitem.asp??l1=2&l2=1&intId=60

MedlinePlus: Asthma
www.nlm.nih.gov/medlineplus/asthma.html

What Is Asthma?
www.nhlbi.nih.gov/health/ dci/Diseases/Asthma/Asthma_WhatIs.
htm

World Health Guide: Asthma in Children
www.worldmedicalguide.com/diseases-and-conditions/ asthma/
asthma-in-children-how-to-tackle-it/

World Health Organization: Asthma
www.who.int/topics/asthma/en/

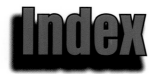

Index

Picture Credits

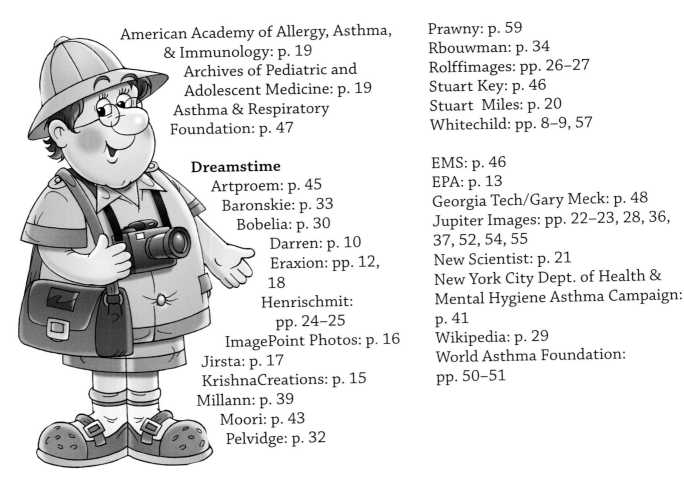

American Academy of Allergy, Asthma, & Immunology: p. 19
Archives of Pediatric and Adolescent Medicine: p. 19
Asthma & Respiratory Foundation: p. 47

Dreamstime
Artproem: p. 45
Baronskie: p. 33
Bobelia: p. 30
Darren: p. 10
Eraxion: pp. 12, 18
Henrischmit: pp. 24–25
ImagePoint Photos: p. 16
Jirsta: p. 17
KrishnaCreations: p. 15
Millann: p. 39
Moori: p. 43
Pelvidge: p. 32

Prawny: p. 59
Rbouwman: p. 34
Rolffimages: pp. 26–27
Stuart Key: p. 46
Stuart Miles: p. 20
Whitechild: pp. 8–9, 57

EMS: p. 46
EPA: p. 13
Georgia Tech/Gary Meck: p. 48
Jupiter Images: pp. 22–23, 28, 36, 37, 52, 54, 55
New Scientist: p. 21
New York City Dept. of Health & Mental Hygiene Asthma Campaign: p. 41
Wikipedia: p. 29
World Asthma Foundation: pp. 50–51

To the best knowledge of the publisher, all other images are in the public domain. If any image has been inadvertently uncredited, please notify Harding House Publishing Service, Vestal, New York 13850, so that rectification can be made for future printings.

About the Author

Rae Simons has written many books for young adults and children.

About the Consultant

Elise DeVore Berlan, MD, MPH, FAAP, is a faculty member of the Division of Adolescent Health at Nationwide Children's Hospital and an Assistant Professor of Clinical Pediatrics at The Ohio State University College of Medicine. She completed her Fellowship in Adolescent Medicine at Children's Hospital Boston and obtained a Master's Degree in Public Health at the Harvard School of Public Health. Dr. Berlan completed her residency in pediatrics at the Children's Hospital of Philadelphia, where she also served an additional year as Chief Resident. She received her medical degree from the University of Iowa College of Medicine.